The L

Book

of Simple

Herbal

Remedies

Discover over 100 herbal Medicine for all kinds
of Ailment.

Inspired By

Barbara O'Neill

Blossom Davis

Copyright © 2023 **Blossom Davis**

Paperback ISBN: 978-1-961902-89-3

Disclaimer:

The information provided in this book is for informational purposes only. Please consult with your health care provider for medical advice. The author specifically disclaims any liability that is incurred from the use or application of the contents of this book

Contents

Introduction to The Lost Book of Herbal Remedies: Rediscovering Nature's Wisdom

In a world where modern medicine dominates, the timeless wisdom of nature often remains hidden, like pages of a forgotten book. "The Lost Book of Herbal Remedies" is an invitation to turn back the clock and rediscover the natural healing power that surrounds us.

Inspired by the teachings of Barbara O'Neill, a renowned advocate for natural health, this book is a testament to the wonders of the plant kingdom. O'Neill, with her deep understanding of holistic health, has long championed the idea that nature offers us not just ingredients for survival, but powerful allies in our journey to wellness.

In these pages, you will embark on an exploratory journey through nature's own pharmacy. From the humble backyard weed to the majestic forest herb, each plant holds secrets waiting to be unlocked. This book is more than a compilation of remedies; it's a bridge to the past, reconnecting us with age-old traditions of healing that were once common knowledge.

Whether you are a novice in the world of herbal remedies or a seasoned herbalist, this book aims to enlighten and inspire. It's not just about learning which plants can heal; it's about fostering a deeper connection with nature and empowering yourself with knowledge that our ancestors held dear.

"The Lost Book of Herbal Remedies" is not merely a guide; it's a journey into the heart of nature's healing power. As Barbara O'Neill has shown us, health is a harmony between body and nature, and this book is your guide to achieving that harmony. Let's turn the pages and rediscover the lost knowledge that can nourish and heal us.

As we delve deeper into "The Lost Book of Herbal Remedies," we uncover a Goldmine of natural solutions, drawing from the profound wisdom of Barbara O'Neill. This chapter is dedicated to unraveling the simple, yet powerful remedies for common illnesses that big pharmaceutical companies often overshadow with their complex, and sometimes unnecessary, treatments.

Understanding the Basics

Before diving into specific remedies, it's crucial to grasp the fundamental principles that underpin Barbara O'Neill's approach:

The Power of Prevention: O'Neill emphasizes that the best remedy is prevention. A diet rich in whole, plant-based foods and an active lifestyle are key.

Listening to Your Body: Understanding the signals your body sends is crucial. Often, symptoms are an indication of deeper imbalances that need addressing.

Common Illnesses and Natural Remedies:

Colds and Flu: Instead of over-the-counter cold medications, try echinacea, elderberry, and ginger tea. These natural remedies boost your immune system and provide relief from symptoms.

Digestive Issues: For indigestion, bloating, and constipation, remedies include peppermint tea, aloe vera juice, and probiotic-rich foods like fermented vegetables.

Skin Conditions: For issues like eczema and acne, natural remedies such as aloe vera, tea tree oil, and turmeric have anti-inflammatory and healing properties.

Stress and Anxiety: Instead of immediately turning to medication for stress, consider natural options like chamomile tea, lavender essential oil, and practicing mindfulness or yoga.

Joint Pain and Inflammation: Remedies such as turmeric (curcumin), ginger, and omega-3 rich foods like flaxseeds can be effective in managing inflammation.

Insomnia: For a better night's sleep, consider valerian root, magnesium-rich foods like almonds, and establishing a calming bedtime routine.

Empowering Yourself

This chapter is not just a list of remedies; it's an empowerment tool. By understanding and utilizing these natural solutions, you take control of your health. Remember, the journey to wellness is as much about nurturing the mind and spirit as it is about treating the body. Let's embrace the wisdom of Barbara O'Neill and rediscover the healing power of nature.

There are several conditions for which herbal treatments have been utilized successfully over the years. These plant-based medicines have been used for thousands of years to improve people's health and well-being. Many common health problems can be treated successfully with herbal medicines, without resorting to harmful chemicals or pharmaceuticals. Because of their low price and quick availability, they are frequently considered as a viable choice. The anti-inflammatory, digestive, immune system-stimulating, and general health benefits of herbal treatments are numerous. Although herbal medicines are all-natural, that doesn't imply they're appropriate for everyone. If you have any preexisting health conditions, are pregnant, or are breastfeeding, you should talk to your doctor before starting any herbal treatment. This article will teach you about the most often used herbal treatments and the conditions they address. You will learn about the various health benefits of herbs, such as ginger for nausea, slippery elm for diarrhea, quercetin for allergies, chamomile for acid reflux, nettle leaf for anemia, and many others.

Acid reflux, commonly known as gastroesophageal reflux disease (GERD), is a common disorder in which stomach acid runs back into the esophagus, generating a burning sensation in the chest or neck. There are some natural therapies that may aid with acid reflux, and they are as follows:

Aloe vera is a natural anti-inflammatory that can help calm your stomach and protect your esophagus from acid.

Baking soda is a common household ingredient that can be used as a natural antacid to help alleviate stomach acid and its associated symptoms.

The saliva produced in response to chewing gum can help neutralize stomach acid and flush it out of the esophagus.

Ginger: Acid reflux symptoms like nausea, vomiting, and stomach pain may find relief with ginger.

Elevating your head and upper body while you sleep can reduce the risk of acid reflux from your stomach entering your esophagus.

Eating more frequently and in smaller portions can help lower stomach acid production.

Avoid certain foods: Certain foods, such as citrus fruits, chocolate, spicy foods, and fatty foods might exacerbate acid reflux symptoms.

Don't smoke or drink alcohol and try to avoid caffeinated drinks

Here are some Remedies you can start using now to Relief you of Most Sickness Known to Man.

Remedies for Acid Reflux

A drink made from aloe vera juice and honey is one acid reflux remedy you can try. Here's a basic recipe for the drink:

Ingredients:

a quarter cup aloe vera juice

1 teaspoon honey

1 cup of water

Instructions:

In a small mixing bowl, combine the aloe vera juice and honey.

Pour a cup of water over the mixture.

To help neutralize stomach acid, drink the mixture slowly about 20 minutes before a meal.

Aloe vera juice can have a strong and sometimes bitter taste; to make it more palatable, dilute it with water or add more honey. You should also be aware that aloe vera latex can cause side effects such as abdominal cramps, diarrhea, dehydration, and electrolyte imbalance, so use aloe vera juice only under the supervision of a healthcare professional.

Remedy 2

Ginger tea

Ingredients:

1 inch ginger root piece

1 quart of water

Instructions:

Ginger root, peeled and grate

Bring one cup of water to a boil, then add the ginger root.

Allow it to simmer for 10 minutes.

Strain the tea and drink it slowly, about 20 minutes before a meal or whenever you experience acid reflux symptoms.

Ginger contains natural anti-inflammatory properties that may aid in esophageal soothing and stomach acid neutralization. If you find the ginger to be too strong, dilute it with honey or lemon juice to taste. As always, consult your healthcare professional before making any dietary changes, and keep in mind that large amounts of ginger may cause stomach discomfort or heartburn.

Remedy 3

A baking soda solution

Ingredients:

half a teaspoon baking soda

half a cup of water

Instructions:

In a small glass, combine the baking soda and water.

Drink the mixture slowly, but keep in mind that baking soda has a high sodium content and should be consumed in moderation and under the supervision of a healthcare professional.

Baking soda is a natural antacid that can help neutralize stomach acid and relieve symptoms of acid reflux. Baking soda solution can also help to neutralize stomach acid and keep it from returning to the esophagus. However, excessive use of baking soda can cause side effects such as gas, bloating, and diarrhea. If you have high blood pressure or kidney disease, you should also limit your sodium intake.

Remedy 4

Tea made with chamomile flowers

What you need:

1 tsp. dried chamomile flowers (optional)

1.25 ounces of water

Instructions:

Put a cup of water on the stove and add a teaspoon of dried chamomile flowers.

Let the tea steep for 5 minutes, then filter.

Intake of the tea should occur once or twice daily.

Chamomile's anti-inflammatory characteristics make it useful for easing the discomfort of acid reflux.

Remedy 5

Cup of tea made from marshmallow roots

Measure out 1 tsp. of dried marshmallow root.

1.25 ounces of water

Instructions:

Put 1 teaspoon of dried marshmallow root into 1 cup of water and bring to a boil.

Let the tea steep for 10 minutes, then strain.

Intake of the tea should occur once or twice daily.

The mucilaginous material found in marshmallow root can coat the stomach and intestines, preventing irritation and alleviating acid reflux symptoms.

Remedy 6

An infusion of licorice root

You'll need 1 teaspoon of dried licorice root.

1.25 ounces of water

Instructions:

Put one teaspoon of dried licorice root into water that has been brought to a boil.

Let the tea steep for 5 minutes, then filter.

Intake of the tea should occur once or twice daily.

In addition to calming the stomach and relieving acid reflux symptoms, licorice root can help increase the mucus coating of the esophagus, making it better able to withstand stomach acid.

Remedy 7

Tea made from dandelion roots

Dandelion root, dry, 1 teaspoon

1.25 ounces of water

Instructions:

Put one teaspoon of dried dandelion root into water that has been brought to a boil.

Let the tea steep for 5 minutes, then filter.

Intake of the tea should occur once or twice daily.

Acid reflux symptoms may be alleviated by using dandelion root, a natural diuretic that also helps with inflammation and digestion.

Remedy 8

Infusion of slippery elm bark

One teaspoon of dried slippery elm bark is the only ingredient needed.

1.25 ounces of water

Instructions:

Bring a cup of water to a boil and add a teaspoon of dried slippery elm bark.

Let the tea steep for 5 minutes, then filter.

Intake of the tea should occur once or twice daily.

Because of its natural mucilaginous characteristics, slipper elm bark can coat the stomach and intestines, creating a barrier against irritants and relieving acid reflux symptoms.

Remedies for Anemia

REMEDY 1

Salad with Spinach and Strawberries

Ingredients

2 cups freshly picked spinach leaves

1 cup strawberries, sliced

1 teaspoon lemon juice

1 teaspoon of honey

Instructions:

Combine the spinach leaves and strawberries in a large mixing bowl.

To make the dressing, combine the lemon juice and honey in a small bowl.

Toss the salad with the dressing to combine.

The salad is high in vitamin C and iron, which can aid in iron absorption and prevent anemia.

Remedy 2:

Beets Juice

Ingredients:

1 beetroot, medium

1 carrot, medium

1 apple

1 quart of water

Instructions:

All vegetables and fruits should be washed and peeled.

Cut the vegetables and fruits into bite-sized pieces.

Blend all of the ingredients in a blender until smooth.

To get the best results, drink the juice right away.

Beets are high in folate, vitamin C, and iron, and beet juice can help boost hemoglobin levels, which can help treat anemia.

Remedy 3

Blackstrap Molasses

Ingredients:

1 tablespoon molasses (blackstrap)

1 cup of hot water

Instructions:

In a cup of warm water, combine the blackstrap molasses.

It should be consumed once a day, before going to bed.

Blackstrap molasses contains iron, which can help increase iron levels in the blood and prevent anemia.

Remedy 4

Nettle Leaf Tea

For a cup of nettle leaf tea, you'll need: 1 teaspoon of dried nettle leaves.

1.25 ounces of water

Instructions:

Put one teaspoon of dried nettle leaves into a pot of water and bring it to a boil.

Let the tea steep for 5 minutes, then filter.

Intake of the tea should occur once or twice daily.

Nettle leaf is useful for preventing and treating anemia since it contains iron, vitamin C, and other elements necessary for the synthesis of red blood cells.

Remedy 5

Culinary beverage brewed from red raspberry leaves

What you'll need:

Red raspberry leaves, 1 teaspoon dried

1.25 ounces of water

Instructions:

In a pot with one cup of water, add one teaspoon of dried red raspberry leaves and bring to a boil.

Let the tea steep for 5 minutes, then filter.

Intake of the tea should occur once or twice daily.

It has been found that the iron and vitamin C found in red raspberry leaves can aid in the prevention and treatment of anemia.

Remedy 6

Juice from spinach

Ingredients:

Fresh spinach leaves, enough for 1 cup

Preparing a glass of juice from fresh spinach leaves requires blending one cup of the leaves.

Have a glass of the juice daily.

Spinach can be used to prevent and treat anemia due to its high iron and nutritional content, both of which are crucial for the body to produce healthy red blood cells.

Remedy 7

Sugarcane molasses with a touch of blackstrap

What You'll Need:

1 tbsp. of Dark Molasses

Blackstrap molasses and water should be mixed at a ratio of 1 tablespoon to 8 ounces.

Take the concoction twice day.

The iron and other nutrients in blackstrap molasses aid in the formation of red blood cells and can be used to treat or prevent anemia.

Remedy 8

Salivary Value of Parsley Extract

Ingredients:

One cup of chopped fresh parsley

One cup of fresh parsley leaves should be blended into a juicer.

Have a glass of the juice daily.

Parsley's high iron and nutritional content makes it a useful tool in the fight against and treatment of anemia.

Remedy 9

Juice Extract from the Beet

Ingredients:

One fresh beetroot (one cup)

In order to prepare beet juice, you will need to blend 1 cup of fresh beets.

Have a glass of the juice daily.

Beetroot's high iron and nutritional content makes it a useful tool in the fight against and treatment of anemia.

Remedies for Diabetes

Remedy 1

Tea made from fenugreek seeds

1 teaspoon dried fenugreek seeds

1 quart of water

Instructions:

Soak 1 teaspoon of fenugreek seeds in 1 cup of water overnight.

In the morning, strain the seeds and drink the water.

Repeat the procedure twice daily.

Fenugreek is well-known for its ability to improve insulin sensitivity and lower blood sugar levels.

Remedy 2

Bitter gourd Juice

Ingredients

1 bitter gourd, chopped

1 quart of water

Instructions

Remove the seeds from the bitter gourd and cut it into pieces.

In a blender, combine the bitter gourd and 1 cup of water.

Drink the juice on an empty stomach after straining it.

Repeat the procedure twice daily.

Bitter gourd contains an insulin-like compound that can aid in insulin sensitivity and blood sugar control.

Remedy 3

Cinnamon Tea

Ingredients:

1 tablespoon cinnamon powder

1 quart of water

Instructions:

Bring 1 cup of water to a boil and add 1 teaspoon cinnamon powder.

After 5 minutes of simmering, strain the tea.

Before meals, drink the tea.

Cinnamon has been shown to help control blood sugar levels.

Remedy 4

Tea made with bitter melon

Ingredients:

To a teaspoon of dried bitter melon

1.25 ounces of water

Instructions:

To prepare, bring a cup of water to a boil and stir in a teaspoon of dried bitter melon.

Let the tea steep for 5 minutes, then filter.

Intake of the tea should occur once or twice daily.

In persons with diabetes, bitter melon has chemicals that have been demonstrated to reduce blood sugar and increase insulin sensitivity.

Remedy 5

Drinking a cup of cinnamon tea

Ingredients:

Mix 1 tsp. of cinnamon powder with 1 cup of sugar

1.25 ounces of water

Instructions:

Prepare a cup of cinnamon water by bringing a teaspoon of cinnamon powder and a cup of water to a boil.

Let the tea steep for 5 minutes, then filter.

Intake of the tea should occur once or twice daily.

People with diabetes who consume cinnamon regularly had lower blood sugar levels and a lower risk of developing diabetic complications.

Remedies for Bloating and gastroenteritis

Remedy 1

Peppermint Tea

Ingredients:

1 tsp. dried peppermint leaves

1 quart of water

Instructions:

Bring 1 cup of water to a boil, then add 1 teaspoon of dried peppermint leaves.

After 5 minutes of simmering, strain the tea.

If you suffer from bloating or abdominal pain, sip some tea whenever you need relief.

Fourth, peppermint's anti-inflammatory qualities can help calm an upset stomach and ease gas.

Remedy 2

Cucumber-Ginger Tea

What You Need:

a One-Inch Section of Ginger Root

1.25 ounces of water

Instructions:

Make ginger powder by combining 1 teaspoon ground ginger with 1 teaspoon sugar

Bring a cup of water to a boil and then add the ginger root.

Simmer for 10 minutes.

Tea should be sipped slowly after being strained.

There are anti-inflammatory qualities in ginger that can help calm an upset stomach and reduce gas.

Remedy 3

Tea Made with Fennel Seeds

What You'll Need:

1 tsp. of fennel seeds

1.25 ounces of water

Instructions:

Put one teaspoon of fennel seeds into a cup of water and bring it to a boil.

Let the tea steep for 5 minutes, then filter.

If you suffer from bloating and abdominal pain, drink the tea as needed.

In addition to its culinary uses, fennel possesses natural carminative qualities that may help alleviate gas and bloating.

It's possible that some people are allergic to, or have negative drug interactions with, particular herbs or foods. Keep in mind that gas and tummy aches could be indicators of anything more serious, so it's important to be checked out by a doctor if you're experiencing them.

Remedies for Problems sleeping/insomnia

Remedy 1

Drinking some passion-inducing passion-flower tea

Ingredients:

1 tsp. of dried passionflower leaves

1.25 ounces of water

Instructions:

Bring a cup of water to a boil and add a teaspoonful of dried passionflower leaves.

Let the tea steep for 5 minutes, then filter.

Try having a cup of tea approximately an hour before bedtime.

Passionflower has natural sedative properties that can help to promote relaxation and improve sleep.

Remedy 2

Drinking some Valerian root tea

Ingredients:

One teaspoon of valerian root powder

1.25 ounces of water

Instructions:

Put a teaspoon of dried valerian root into a cup of boiling water.

Let the tea steep for 10 minutes, then strain.

Try having a cup of tea approximately an hour before bedtime.

The use of valerian root, which contains naturally occurring sedative qualities, has been shown to aid with relaxing and sleep quality.

Remedy 3

Cup of skullcap

Ingredients:

Dried skullcap leaves, one teaspoon

1.25 ounces of water

Instructions:

Prepare a cup of skullcap tea by bringing a teaspoon of dried leaves to a boil in a cup of water.

Let the tea steep for 5 minutes, then filter.

Try having a cup of tea approximately an hour before bedtime.

There are natural sedative properties in skullcap that might aid in relaxation and make it easier to drift off to sleep.

Remedy 4

Medicinal Chamomile Tea

Ingredients:

One teaspoon of chamomile blossoms

1.25 ounces of water

Instructions:

Put a cup of water on the stove and add a teaspoon of dried chamomile flowers.

Let the tea steep for 5 minutes, then filter.

Take the tea about an hour before you plan to hit the hay.

The calming and sleep-inducing effects of chamomile come from its natural sedative qualities.

Remedy 5

Herbal Infusion with Valerian Root

Ingredients:

1/2 gram of kava kava root

1.25 ounces of water

Instructions:

To prepare, bring a cup of water and a teaspoon of valerian root to a boil.

Let the tea steep for 10 minutes, then strain.

Try having a cup of tea approximately an hour before bedtime.

As a natural sedative, valerian root can aid in stress reduction and quality slumber.

Remedy 6

Oil of Lavender

Lavender essential oil, 1–2 drops

The recommended amount of lavender essential oil to put into a diffuser or a bowl of water is 1-2 drops.

Try sniffing the scent from a basin of water or setting up a diffuser next to your bed.

Try it out around an hour before bed, or anytime you think it might help you unwind and get better rest.

Due to its innate sedative characteristics, lavender is often used to aid with restful sleep.

Remedies for Eyes pain

Remedy 1

Cucumber Cuts

The recipe calls for one cucumber.

Thinly slice a cucumber, as directed.

Laid back with the cucumbers over your eyes, you can relax.

The cucumber slices should be left on for about 15 to 20 minutes.

The anti-inflammatory and antioxidant properties of cucumber make it an effective treatment for under-the-eye puffiness.

Remedy 2

The Benefits of a Warm Compress

Preparation calls just one dish of hot water.

A single, spotless washcloth

Instructions:

Wring out a fresh washcloth in some hot water.

Put the damp washcloth over your closed eyes and squeeze away the excess water.

Ten to fifteen minutes of heat application is recommended.

Do this a couple of times a day, every day.

Reduce eye puffiness and relax tired eyes with a warm compress.

Remedy 3:

Exercises for the Eyes

Directions:

Keep your back straight and sit in a position of comfort.

For a few seconds, try fixing your gaze on something in the room without moving your head.

Try closing your eyes and imagining what it looks like.

Take a few seconds to gently blink your eyes back and forth, up and down, and all about.

To unwind your eyes, simply blink several times.

Do this routine twice or thrice a day.

Strengthening the eye muscles, increasing blood flow, and relieving stress on the eyes can all be accomplished by regular eye training.

If you have allergies, are pregnant, or breastfeeding, you should talk to a doctor before using essential oils. As with any symptom or disease, it's best to consult a doctor if your eyes continue to bother you or if you suspect you may have an underlying problem.

Remedy 4

Eyebright tea

Ingredients

1 teaspoon of dried eyebright herb

1.25 ounces of water

Instructions:

Put a spoonful of dried eyebright herb into a cup of boiling water.

Let the tea steep for 5 minutes, then filter.

Indulge in a cup of tea at room temperature.

Tea bags can be cooled and used to compress a clean washcloth, which you can then drape over your closed eyelids.

Ten to fifteen minutes is plenty of time to let the compress do its job.

The recommended frequency is twice or thrice each day.

It has been found that the anti-inflammatory chemicals found in eyebright can help reduce puffiness and relieve irritation around the eyes.

Remedy 5

Tea made with bilberries

Ingredients:

a single teaspoon of bilberry leaves, dried

1.25 ounces of water

Instructions:

Put one teaspoon of dried bilberry leaves into a cup of boiling water.

Let the tea steep for 5 minutes, then filter.

One cup of tea each day is recommended.

Boosting circulation to the eyes and lowering the likelihood of eye disorders are two of the many benefits associated with consuming bilberry.

Remedy 6

Cup of ginkgo biloba

One teaspoon of dried ginkgo biloba leaves is the main ingredient.

1.25 ounces of water

Instructions:

Prepare a ginkgo biloba tea by bringing one cup of water to a boil and adding one teaspoon of dried leaves.

Let the tea steep for 5 minutes, then filter.

Take the tea daily, once.

In studies, Ginkgo Biloba was found to increase blood flow to the eyes and protect against age-related macular degeneration.

Some herbs may have negative interactions with prescribed drugs, and others may simply not be appropriate for some persons. If you have any preexisting health conditions, are pregnant, or are breastfeeding, you should talk to your doctor before starting any herbal treatment.

Remedies for Kidney

Remedy 1

Cup of dandelions

Ingredients:

1 tsp. of dandelion root, dried

1.25 ounces of water

Instructions:

Put 1 teaspoon of dried dandelion root into 1 cup of boiling water.

Let the tea steep for 10 minutes, then strain.

Take the tea daily, once.

Natural diuretic qualities found in dandelion root may support healthy kidney function and eliminate waste products.

Remedy 2

Herbal infusion flavored with parsley

Ingredients

Parsley leaves, dried, one teaspoon

1.25 ounces of water

Instructions:

Prepare by bringing 1 cup of water to a boil and stirring in 1 teaspoon of dried parsley leaves.

Let the tea steep for 5 minutes, then filter.

Take the tea daily, once.

The natural diuretic in parsley can boost kidney health and eliminate waste products.

Remedy 3
Medicinal horsetail infusion

Ingredients:

Horsetail herb, dried, one teaspoon

1.25 ounces of water

Instructions:

To make, bring a cup of water to a boil and stir in 1

Remedy 4
Fruit juice made from cranberries

Ingredients:

Cranberry juice, one cup

Combine 1 cup of cranberry juice with 8 ounces of water, according to the instructions.

Take the concoction twice day.

Antioxidants and other substances found in abundance in cranberry juice have been shown to be effective in warding off and treating kidney infections and possibly even lowering the likelihood of developing kidney stones.

Remedy 5

Cup of dandelions

Dandelion leaves, dried, one teaspoon

1.25 ounces of water

Instructions:

Put one teaspoon of dried dandelion leaves into water that has been brought to a boil.

Let the tea steep for 5 minutes, then filter.

Intake of the tea should occur once or twice daily.

Toxins are eliminated and renal health is enhanced by dandelion's diuretic properties.

Remedies for Arthritis

Remedy 1

Cup of tumeric-infused tea

Ingredients:

Mix 1 tsp. of turmeric powder with 1 tsp.

1.25 ounces of water

Instructions:

Combine 1 teaspoon of turmeric powder with 1 cup of boiling water.

Let the tea steep for 5 minutes, then filter.

You should have the tea once or twice a day.

Arthritis joint pain and inflammation can be alleviated by turmeric's anti-inflammatory effects.

Remedy 2

The Devil's Claw

Ingredients:

Dried devil's claw root, one teaspoon

1.25 ounces of water

Instructions:

Bring a cup of water to a boil and add a teaspoon of dried devil's claw root.

Let the tea steep for 10 minutes, then strain.

Intake of the tea should occur once or twice daily.

Traditional herbal medicine has long relied on devil's claw to alleviate the discomfort and swelling of arthritic joints.

Remedy 3

Ginger tea

What You Need:

A One-Inch Section of Ginger Root

1.25 ounces of water

Instructions:

Make ginger powder by combining 1 teaspoon ground ginger with 1 teaspoon sugar

Bring a cup of water to a boil and then add the ginger root.

Simmer for 10 minutes.

Tea should be sipped slowly after being strained.

Having anti-inflammatory qualities, ginger can help alleviate arthritis-related joint pain and swelling.

Remedies for Skin Care

Remedy 1
Aloe vera juice
What you need:

One aloe vera leaf is the only required ingredient.

Instructions:

Prepare aloe vera gel by slicing up a leaf.

Put the gel on the irritated skin.

For 20-30 minutes, let it run.

Clear it with with water.

A natural moisturizer with anti-inflammatory characteristics, aloe vera gel can help calm and heal the skin.

Remedy 2
Calendula oil
Ingredient:

Calendula petals, about a quarter cup

One-half cup of base oil (such as coconut or jojoba oil)

Instructions:

Carrier oil should be heated in a double boiler or a heatproof dish placed over a saucepan of gently simmering water.

After the oil has warmed, add the calendula petals and mix well.

For 30–40 minutes, stirring regularly, warm the mixture on low heat to infuse the oil with the herb.

Put the oil through a strainer and then into an airtight container.

There are anti-inflammatory components in calendula oil that can aid in the healing process.

Remedy 3

Mask Made From Green Tea

What you need:

One bag of green tea, sugar, and milk.

Only one-fourth of a cup of water

Instructions:

Prepare some ice for your cup of green tea.

Tea leaves can be accessed by slicing apart a tea bag.

To make a paste, combine the leaves with a quarter cup of water.

Face mask time: 15-20 minutes after applying the paste.

Take a shower and dry it off with a towel.

Antioxidants in green tea help prevent skin damage and inflammation, resulting in a more radiant and young appearance.

Remedies for Migraine/Headaches

Remedy 1

Herbal tea made from feverfew

Ingredients:

a single teaspoon of feverfew leaves, dried

1.25 ounces of water

Instructions:

Put one teaspoon of dried feverfew leaves into a cup of boiling water.

Let the tea steep for 5 minutes, then filter.

Take the tea daily, once.

Feverfew's anti-inflammatory qualities can help lessen the severity and frequency of migraine attacks.

Remedy 2

Cup of butterbur

Ingredients:

1/2 ounce of fresh butterbur root

1.25 ounces of water

Instructions:

In a pot of boiling water, steep 1 teaspoon of dried butterbur root for a minute.

Let the tea steep for 10 minutes, then strain.

You should have the tea at least twice a day.

Migraine attacks and their severity can be mitigated with the use of butterbur.

Remedy 3

Medicinal use of peppermint oil

What you need:

Two to three drops of pure peppermint oil.

Instructions:

Blend with a carrier oil and rub onto your temples and the back of your neck, or use a diffuser.

Take a deep breath of the fragrance, or give yourself a soothing massage.

The natural pain-relieving qualities of peppermint oil make it useful for alleviating headaches and migraines.

Furthermore, it is best to seek expert help if your symptoms persist or worsen.

Remedies for Anxiety and depression

Remedy 1

Tea with lemon balm

What you need

Dried lemon balm leaves, 1 teaspoon

1.25 ounces of water

Instructions:

Bring a cup of water to a boil and add a teaspoon of dried lemon balm leaves.

Let the tea steep for 5 minutes, then filter.

Intake of the tea should occur once or twice daily.

The natural sedative effects of lemon balm make it an attractive treatment for anxiety and stress.

Remedy 2

Drinking some passion-inducing passion-flower tea

Ingredients:

1 tsp. of dried passionflower leaves

1.25 ounces of water

Instructions:

Bring a cup of water to a boil and add a teaspoonful of dried passionflower leaves.

Let the tea steep for 5 minutes, then filter.

Intake of the tea should occur once or twice daily.

The passionflower plant has been used for centuries for its relaxing effects on both the mind and body.

Remedy 3

Cup of skullcap

Ingredients:

Dried skullcap leaves, one teaspoon

1.25 ounces of water

Instructions:

Prepare a cup of skullcap tea by bringing a teaspoon of dried leaves to a boil in a cup of water.

Let the tea steep for 5 minutes, then filter.

Intake of the tea should occur once or twice daily.

Skullcap's natural sedative effects aid in the management of stress and the promotion of general well-being.

Remedies for Yeast Infection

Remedy 1

Steeped garlic

Ingredients

Two or three garlic cloves

1.25 ounces of water

Instructions:

Add two or three peeled and crushed cloves of garlic to a cup of water and bring to a boil.

Let the tea steep for 5 minutes, then filter.

Intake of the tea should occur once or twice daily.

The antifungal qualities of garlic make it useful for treating yeast infections.

Remedy 2

Extract from tea trees

Ingredients

Two or three drops of tea tree oil

Tea tree oil should be diluted in a carrier oil like coconut or jojoba oil before use.

Second, using a cotton swab or cotton ball, dab the solution onto the affected region.

Let it sit for 15 to 20 minutes, then wash it off.

Step four: do this thrice a day.

5 Tea tree oil's antifungal qualities can aid in the treatment of yeast infections.

Remedy 3

Yogurt

Ingredients:

plain unsweetened yogurt

Instructions:

Use a cotton swab or cotton ball to apply plain, unsweetened yogurt to the region.

Rinse it off with water after it has been on for around fifteen to twenty minutes.

Do this thrice a day, every day.

Probiotics found in yogurt are good for you and can fight yeast infections and help restore your body's natural bacterial balance.

Once again, some of these treatments may not be appropriate for everyone, or they may interact negatively with other medications. If you have any pre-existing health conditions, are pregnant, or are breastfeeding, you should talk to your doctor before starting any herbal treatment. Furthermore, it is best to seek expert help if your symptoms persist or worsen.

Remedies for Herpes & Cold Sores

Remedy 1

Tea with lemon balm

What you need:

Dried lemon balm leaves, 1 teaspoon

1.25 ounces of water

Instructions:

Bring a cup of water to a boil and add a teaspoon of dried lemon balm leaves.

Let the tea steep for 5 minutes, then filter.

Intake of the tea should occur once or twice daily.

Herpes and cold sore breakouts can be mitigated with the help of lemon balm's antiviral capabilities.

Drinking a cup of licorice root tea

You'll need 1 teaspoon of dried licorice root.

1.25 ounces of water

Instructions:

Put one teaspoon of dried licorice root into water that has been brought to a boil.

Let the tea steep for 10 minutes, then strain.

Intake of the tea should occur once or twice daily.

Herpes and cold sore breakouts can be mitigated with the use of licorice root's anti-inflammatory and antiviral qualities.

Remedy 2

Olive oil concentrate

Capsules of olive leaf extract

Take olive leaf extract capsules as directed on the packaging or as directed by your doctor.

The antiviral characteristics of olive leaf extract can lessen the impact of herpes and cold sore outbreaks.

Remedies for Nerve Repair

Remedy 1

a cup of St. John's Wort tea

What you need:

1 teaspoon of dried St. John's Wort leaves

1.25 ounces of water

Instructions:

Put one teaspoon of dried St. John's Wort leaves into a pot of boiling water.

Let the tea steep for 5 minutes, then filter.

Intake of the tea should occur once or twice daily.

There is a long history of using St. John's Wort for its anti-inflammatory and nerve-repairing effects.

Remedy 2

Cup of tumeric-infused tea

Ingredients:

Mix 1 tsp. of turmeric powder with 1 tsp.

1.25 ounces of water

Instructions:

Combine 1 teaspoon of turmeric powder with 1 cup of boiling water.

Let the tea steep for 5 minutes, then filter.

Intake of the tea should occur once or twice daily.

Curcumin, found in turmeric, is an anti-inflammatory that has been shown to aid with nerve healing and lessen pain.

Remedy 3

Fish oil capsules

Comprised of: Omega-3 Supplements

Instructions: Take Omega-3 supplements as directed on the label or as prescribed by a physician.

Among their many benefits, omega-3 fatty acids are particularly useful for reducing inflammation and supporting normal nerve function.

Remedies for The Heart

Remedy 1

Hawthorn berry infusion

Ingredients:

1/2 a fresh hawthorn berry

1.25 ounces of water

Instructions:

To prepare, bring one cup of water to a boil and stir in one teaspoon of dried hawthorn berries.

Let the tea steep for 10 minutes, then strain.

Intake of the tea should occur once or twice daily.

The hawthorn berry has a history of being utilized to aid the heart and blood vessels.

Remedy 2

Steeped garlic

Ingredients

Two or three garlic cloves

1.25 ounces of water

Instructions:

Add two or three peeled and crushed cloves of garlic to a cup of water and bring to a boil.

Let the tea steep for 5 minutes, then filter.

Intake of the tea should occur once or twice daily.

Historically, garlic has been utilized to promote heart health, reduce blood pressure, and lower cholesterol.

Remedy 3

Tea made from guggul tree resin

Ingredients:

guggul resin, one teaspoon

1.25 ounces of water

Instructions:

Put one teaspoon of guggul resin into a cup of boiling water.

Let the tea steep for 10 minutes, then strain.

Intake of the tea should occur once or twice daily.

Guggul has a long history of traditional use to promote cardiovascular health and reduce cholesterol.

Remedy 4

Garlic dietary supplements

Supplemental garlic

Instructions: Follow the label's dosage recommendation for the garlic supplement.

By enhancing circulation and decreasing inflammation, garlic has been demonstrated to help reduce blood pressure and the risk of developing heart disease.

Remedy 5

Omega-3 fatty acid fish oil supplements

Toppings: Fish oil capsules

Follow the label's dosage recommendations while using a fish oil supplement.

Fish oil's high concentration of omega-3 fatty acids has been linked to positive effects on inflammation, lipid profiles, and cardiovascular health.

Remedies for Fever

Remedy 1

Infusion of elderberries

Ingredients:

1 tsp. of dried elderberries

1.25 ounces of water

Instructions:

Prepare a cup of elderberry tea by bringing a spoonful of dried berries and a cup of water to a boil.

Let the tea steep for 10 minutes, then strain.

Intake of the tea should occur once or twice daily.

The natural antiviral properties of elderberry can help lower fever intensity and duration.

Remedy 2

A cup of yarrow tea

Ingredients:

Yarrow leaves, dry, one teaspoon

1.25 ounces of water

Instructions:

To prepare a cup of yarrow tea, bring a teaspoon's worth of dried leaves to a boil in a cup of water.

Let the tea steep for 5 minutes, then filter.

Intake of the tea should occur once or twice daily.

Yarrow's anti-inflammatory effects make it useful for treating fever and the associated body aches.

Remedy 3

Tea with peppermint

Ingredients:

Peppermint leaves, dried, one teaspoon

1.25 ounces of water

Instructions:

Put a cup of water on the stove and a teaspoon of dried peppermint leaves in it.

Let the tea steep for 5 minutes, then filter.

You should have the tea at least twice a day.

To bring down a high body temperature and alleviate a fever, peppermint can be used for its natural cooling effects.

Remedies for U.T.I

Here are the Remedies for U.T.I ((Urinary Tract Infection) (Urinary Tract Infection)

Remedy 1

Cup of dandelions

What you need:

Dandelion leaves, dried, one teaspoon

1.25 ounces of water

Instructions:

Put one teaspoon of dried dandelion leaves into water that has been brought to a boil.

Let the tea steep for 5 minutes, then filter.

Intake of the tea should occur once or twice daily.

Dandelion's diuretic characteristics aid in the removal of bacteria from the urinary tract, reducing the severity of UTI symptoms.

Remedy 2

Fruit juice made from cranberries

Cranberry juice is the main ingredient.

Drink one or two cups of cranberry juice daily, preferably the unsweetened variety.

The antibacterial characteristics of cranberry juice aid in the removal of bacteria from the urinary tract, hence lowering the risk of UTIs.

Remedy 3

The Benefits of Uva Ursi Tea

Uva ursi leaves, dry, 1 teaspoon

1.25 ounces of water

Instructions:

Put one teaspoon of dried uva ursi leaves into water that has been brought to a boil.

Let the tea steep for 10 minutes, then strain.

Intake of the tea should occur once or twice daily.

With its natural antibacterial characteristics, uva ursi can aid in the removal of bacteria from the urinary system, reducing the severity of a UTI's symptoms.

Remedies For Constipation

Remedy 1

Caffeinated Psyllium Husk Tea

Ingredients:

A single teaspoon of psyllium husk

1.25 ounces of water

Instructions:

Prepare a psyllium husk elixir by bringing one cup of water to a boil and stirring in one teaspoon.

Let the tea steep for 5 minutes, then filter.

Intake of the tea should occur once or twice daily.

The fiber in psyllium husk has been shown to ease constipation and encourage regular bowel movements.

Remedy 2

Primrose Extract

Prune Juice Is An Ingredient.

Take 1 to 2 cups of prune juice daily.

The natural sugars in prune juice can be helpful in stimulating the intestines and facilitating bowel motions.

Remedy 3

Infusion of flaxseed

Here's what you'll need: a single teaspoon of flaxseed

1.25 ounces of water

One teaspoon of flaxseed should be added to a cup of water that has been brought to a boil.

Let the tea steep for 5 minutes, then filter.

Intake of the tea should occur once or twice daily.

Constipation can be alleviated and regular bowel movements can be encouraged thanks to the fiber and mucilage found in flax seed.

Once again, Herbal supplements should be used with caution, and a doctor should be consulted before use if you have any preexisting conditions, are expecting or nursing, or are otherwise not in good health. In the case of a UTI, in particular, it is best to seek expert guidance if your symptoms persist or increase, as the infection must be treated immediately to prevent further consequences.

Remedies For Prostatitis

Remedy 1

The benefits of saw palmetto infusion

Ingredients:

Saw palmetto berries, one teaspoonful

1.25 ounces of water

Instructions:

Put one teaspoon of dried saw palmetto berries into a cup of water and bring it to a boil.

Let the tea steep for 10 minutes, then strain.

Intake of the tea should occur once or twice daily.

Anti-inflammatory qualities in saw palmetto make it useful for treating prostatitis.

Remedy 2

Infusion of stinging nettles

What You'll Need: 1 tsp. of dried nettle leaves

1.25 ounces of water

Instructions:

Put one teaspoon of dried nettle leaves into a pot of water and bring it to a boil.

Let the tea steep for 5 minutes, then filter.

Intake of the tea should occur once or twice daily.

It has been found that the anti-inflammatory qualities of nettle can help reduce inflammation in the prostate and alleviate symptoms of prostatitis.

Remedy 3

Tea made from pygeum bark

Ingredients:

One teaspoon of pygeum bark, dried

1.25 ounces of water

Instructions:

To prepare, bring a cup of water and a teaspoon of dried pygeum bark to a boil.

Let the tea steep for 10 minutes, then strain.

Intake of the tea should occur once or twice daily.

With its anti-inflammatory characteristics, pygeum bark can help reduce prostate inflammation and alleviate the pain and discomfort of prostatitis.

Remedies For Bad breath

Remedy 1

Té de cloves

What You'll Need: 1 tsp. of dried cloves

1.25 ounces of water

Instructions:

Bring a cup of water to a boil and stir in a teaspoon of dried cloves.

Let the tea steep for 5 minutes, then filter.

Intake of the tea should occur once or twice daily.

Clove's natural antiseptic and antibacterial characteristics aid in killing the bacteria that cause foul breath and also help to freshen the breath.

Remedy 2

Fennel seed tea

What you need:

One teaspoon of dried fennel seeds.

1.25 ounces of water

Instructions:

Bring a cup of water to a boil, then sprinkle in a teaspoon of dried fennel seeds.

Let the tea steep for 5 minutes, then filter.

Intake of the tea should occur once or twice daily.

Fennel's antibacterial capabilities help destroy the microorganisms that cause bad breath, while also helping to freshen the breath.

Remedy 3

Herbal infusion flavored with parsley

What you need:

Parsley leaves, dried, one teaspoon

1.25 ounces of water

Instructions:

Put one teaspoon of dried parsley leaves into a pot of boiling water.

Let the tea steep for 5 minutes, then filter.

Intake of the tea should occur once or twice daily.

Parsley's antibacterial abilities can help eliminate the bacteria that cause foul breath, while also leaving the breath smelling fresh and minty.

It's worth noting that not all of these treatments are created equal.

Remedies For Burns

Remedy 1

Aloe vera juice

It contains aloe vera gel as an active ingredient.

Instructions:

Rub some aloe vera gel into the sore spot.

Turn it on and let it run for about a quarter of an hour.

Do this a couple of times a day, every day.

Burns can benefit from aloe vera gel's anti-inflammatory and therapeutic capabilities.

Remedy 2

Infusion of comfrey

What you'll need:

Dried comfrey leaves, 1 teaspoon

1.25 ounces of water

Instructions:

Put one teaspoon of dried comfrey leaves into a pot of boiling water.

Let the tea steep for 5 minutes, then filter.

When the tea has cooled, apply it to the sore spot.

Burns can benefit from comfrey's natural anti-inflammatory and healing capabilities.

Remedy 3

Culinary Uses for Calendula Flowers

Ingredients:

About 1 tsp of dried calendula blossoms

1.25 ounces of water

Instructions:

Bring a cup of water to a boil and stir in a teaspoon of dried calendula flowers.

Let the tea steep for 5 minutes, then filter.

The tea should be cooled before being applied to the skin.

Burns can benefit from calendula's natural anti-inflammatory and healing capabilities.

Remedies For Diarrhea

Remedy 1

Chamomile tea

Ingredients for 1 teaspoon of chamomile tea: dried flowers

1.25 ounces of water

Instructions:

Put a cup of water on the stove and add a teaspoon of dried chamomile flowers.

Let the tea steep for 5 minutes, then filter.

Intake of the tea should occur once or twice daily.

It has been found that the anti-inflammatory effects of chamomile assist to calm the digestive tract and reduce diarrheal symptoms.

Remedy 2

Slipper Elm tea

Ingredients:

One teaspoon of dried slippery elm bark is the only ingredient needed.

1.25 ounces of water

Instructions:

Bring a cup of water to a boil and add a teaspoon of dried slippery elm bark.

Let the tea steep for 10 minutes, then strain.

Intake of the tea should occur once or twice daily.

The gel-like material found in Slipper Elm coats the stomach and intestines, protecting them from irritants and potentially alleviating diarrhea symptoms.

Remedy 3

Ginger tea

What You'll need:

Grated Ginger, 1 teaspoon

1.25 ounces of water

Instructions:

Put one teaspoon of grated ginger into a cup of water and bring it to a boil.

Let the tea steep for 5 minutes, then filter.

Intake of the tea should occur once or twice daily.

Ginger's anti-inflammatory characteristics make it an effective treatment for gastrointestinal issues like nausea, vomiting, and diarrhea.

Remedies For Allergies

Remedy 1

Tea with quercetin

You'll need:

1 tsp. of dried herbs high in quercetin, such onion or capers

1.25 ounces of water

Instructions:

To make a tea high in quercetin, boil a cup of water and stir in a teaspoon of dry herbs like onion or capers.

Let the tea steep for 5 minutes, then filter.

Intake of the tea should occur once or twice daily.

Due to its antihistamine properties, quercetin can help alleviate allergy symptoms like sneezing, watery eyes, and a scratchy throat.

Remedy 2

Cup of butterbur

Ingredients

A single teaspoon of dried butterbur root

1.25 ounces of water

Instructions:

Put 1 teaspoon of dried butterbur root into a pot of water that has been brought to a boil.

Let the tea steep for 10 minutes, then strain.

Intake of the tea should occur once or twice daily.

The common allergy symptoms of sneezing, a runny nose, and itchy eyes have long been treated with butterbur.

Remedy 3

Brewing some bromelain tea

For this recipe, you will need: 1 teaspoon of dried pineapple or papaya herbs high in bromelain

1.25 ounces of water

Instructions:

Bring a cup of water to a boil and add a pinch of dried herbs that are rich in bromelain, like those found in pineapples or papayas.

Let the tea steep for 5 minutes, then filter.

Intake of the tea should occur once or twice daily.

Allergy symptoms including sneezing, a runny nose, and itching can be alleviated with the help of bromelain, a natural anti-inflammatory enzyme.

Remedies For Food Poisoning

Remedy 1

Steeped garlic

What you'll need:

Two or three garlic cloves

1.25 ounces of water

Instructions:

Add two or three peeled and crushed cloves of garlic to a cup of water and bring to a boil.

Let the tea steep for 5 minutes, then filter.

Intake of the tea should occur once or twice daily.

Food poisoning infections can be combated with the use of garlic's natural antibiotic capabilities.

Remedy 2

Cup of tumeric-infused tea

Ingredients:

Mix 1 tsp. of turmeric powder with 1 tsp.

1.25 ounces of water

Instructions:

Combine 1 teaspoon of turmeric powder with 1 cup of boiling water.

Let the tea steep for 5 minutes, then filter.

Intake of the tea should occur once or twice daily.

Natural anti-inflammatory and antioxidant properties in turmeric can alleviate food poisoning symptoms including swelling and pain.

Remedy 3

Tea made with activated charcoal Ingredients

What you'll need:

A powdered form of activated charcoal, one teaspoon

1.25 ounces of water

Instructions:

To prepare, bring a cup of water to a boil and stir in 1 teaspoon of activated charcoal powder.

Mix everything together and set it aside to cool.

Intake of the tea should occur once or twice daily.

Toxins and chemicals that may be the source of your food poisoning can be soaked up by activated charcoal.

Remedies For Toothache

Remedy 1

Oil of clove

What you'll need

The active ingredient is clove oil.

Instructions:

Apply some clove oil to the tooth with a cotton swab, as directed.

Do not remove the oil too soon.

Do this a couple of times a day, every day.

Clove oil's anti-inflammatory and pain-relieving characteristics make it a useful remedy for a toothache.

Remedy 2

Tea with peppermint

Ingredients:

Peppermint leaves, dried, one teaspoon

1.25 ounces of water

Instructions:

Bring a cup of water and a teaspoon of dried peppermint leaves to a boil.

Let the tea steep for 5 minutes, then filter.

When the tea is cool, use it as a mouthwash.

Peppermint possesses anti-inflammatory and pain-relieving qualities that can help alleviate a toothache.

Remedy 3

Guava leaves

The recipe calls for two or three Guava leaves.

To treat a toothache, you should crush two or three guava leaves and lay them on the tooth.

Wait a few minutes before removing the leaves.

Do this a couple of times a day, every day.

The anti-inflammatory and analgesic chemicals found in guava leaves can alleviate the discomfort of a toothache.

Remedies For Earache

Remedy 1

Put few drops of garlic oil in your ear.

Amount: 3 garlic cloves

One-fourth cup of olive oil

Instructions:

Three peeled and crushed garlic cloves should be added to a quarter cup of olive oil.

Warm it up for 5 minutes on low heat.

Then, strain the liquid and set it aside to cool.

Put two or three drops of the garlic oil into your ear using a dropper.

When used topically, garlic oil has been shown to alleviate earache pain and protect against bacterial infections.

Remedy 2

Eardrops infused with mullein oil

Dry mullein flowers, about a quarter cup

A quarter cup of olive oil

Instructions:

Put a quarter cup of dried mullein flowers in a quarter cup of olive oil and warm the mixture slowly for 5 minutes.

Then, strain the liquid and set it aside to cool.

Put two or three drops of the mullein oil in your ear using a dropper.

Due to its anti-inflammatory characteristics, mullein oil can alleviate earache pain and swelling.

Remedy 3

Ear drops made with colloidal silver

Colloidal silver is used.

Using a dropper, place two to three drops of colloidal silver in the afflicted ear.

Do this a couple of times a day, every day.

Because of its antibacterial characteristics, colloidal silver can be used to treat earaches and prevent infections.

Remedies For High Blood Pressure

Remedy 1

Tea made with hibiscus petals

Ingredients:

Dried hibiscus flowers, one teaspoon

1.25 ounces of water

Instructions:

Prepare a cup of hibiscus tea by bringing a spoonful of dried flowers and one cup of water to a boil.

Let the tea steep for 5 minutes, then filter.

Intake of the tea should occur once or twice daily.

The traditional usage of hibiscus has been to reduce hypertension and boost cardiovascular health.

Remedy 2

Tea made from celery seeds

What You'll Need:

1 tsp. of celery seeds

1.25 ounces of water

Instructions:

Put a teaspoon of celery seeds in a cup of boiling water.

Let the tea steep for 5 minutes, then filter.

Intake of the tea should occur once or twice daily.

The natural diuretic in celery seed may help reduce blood pressure by eliminating excess fluid in the body.

Remedy 3

Cup of hawthorn berry tea

Ingredients:

1/2 a fresh hawthorn berry

1.25 ounces of water

Instructions:

To prepare, bring one cup of water to a boil and stir in one teaspoon of dried hawthorn berries.

Let the tea steep for 5 minutes, then filter.

Intake of the tea should occur once or twice daily.

The hawthorn fruit has a long history of traditional use for its beneficial effects on cardiovascular health, including its ability to reduce blood pressure through the dilation of blood vessels and strengthening of the heart muscle.

Remedy 4

Supplements made from celery seeds

Nutritional supplement made from celery seeds

Instructions: Follow the label's dosage recommendations for the celery seed supplement you're using.

Compounds in celery seed have been proven to have beneficial effects on blood pressure and circulation.

Remedy 5

Taking Coenzyme Q10 supplements

Supplemental Coenzyme Q10

Follow the dosing recommendations on the bottle of your Coenzyme Q10 supplement.

The antioxidant properties of coenzyme Q10 have been found to benefit heart health and reduce blood pressure.

Remedies For ADHD/ADD

Remedy 1

Tea made from ginkgo biloba leaves

What you'll need:

One teaspoon of dried ginkgo biloba leaves is the main ingredient.

1.25 ounces of water

Instructions:

Bring a cup of water to a boil, then add a teaspoon of dried ginkgo biloba leaves.

Let the tea steep for 5 minutes, then filter.

Intake of the tea should occur once or twice daily.

There is some evidence that the herb ginkgo biloba, which has long been used to boost memory and cognition, can also alleviate the symptoms of attention deficit hyperactivity disorder (ADHD).

Remedy 2

A Cup of Bacopa Monnieri

Ingredients:

Dissolve 1 teaspoon of dried Bacopa monnieri leaves in a cup of water.

1.25 ounces of water

Instructions:

Put one teaspoon of dried Bacopa monnieri leaves into a pot of boiling water.

Let the tea steep for 5 minutes, then filter.

Intake of the tea should occur once or twice daily.

Bacopa monnieri is a herb that has been used for centuries to boost memory and focus and that shows promise for alleviating some ADHD/ADD symptoms.

Remedy 3

The health benefits of Gotu Kola tea

Ingredients

Gotu kola leaf, dry, one teaspoon

1.25 ounces of water

Instructions:

Simply bring a cup of water to a boil and stir in a teaspoon of dried Gotu Kola leaves.

Let the tea steep for 5 minutes, then filter.

Intake of the tea should occur once or twice daily.

Gotu kola is a herbal supplement commonly used to enhance memory and focus, and it has been linked to fewer ADHD/ADD symptoms.

Remedy 4

Tee with Lemon Balm

Dried lemon balm leaves, 1 teaspoon

1.25 ounces of water

Instructions:

Bring a cup of water to a boil and add a teaspoon of dried lemon balm leaves.

Let the tea steep for 5 minutes, then filter.

Intake of the tea should occur once or twice daily.

As a traditional remedy for low spirits, lemon balm may also alleviate some of the negative effects of ADHD by calming the mind and body.

Some of these treatments may not be appropriate for everyone, or they may interact negatively with other medications. If you have any pre-existing health conditions, are pregnant, or are breastfeeding, you should talk to your doctor before starting any herbal treatment. It's also worth noting that ADHD is a multifaceted condition with substantial individual variation in both its causes and responses to treatment. Some people have reported that using herbal supplements for ADHD has helped with symptoms, however it is unclear whether or not these supplements actually treat the underlying cause of the disorder. Therefore, it is crucial to get a comprehensive diagnosis and treatment plan from a skilled healthcare practitioner if you or your child exhibits symptoms of ADHD.

Conclusion

In conclusion, traditional herbal treatments have been utilized to treat a wide range of conditions for millennia. Ginger for motion sickness, slippery elm for diarrhea, quercetin for allergies, garlic oil for earaches, hibiscus tea for hypertension, and ginkgo biloba, Bacopa monnieri, and Gotu Kola for attention deficit hyperactivity disorder are all common herbal treatments.

Remember that these treatments could potentially conflict with your current drugs, and that they might not be appropriate for everyone. If you have any preexisting health conditions, are pregnant, or are breastfeeding, you should talk to your doctor before starting any herbal treatment. Furthermore, it is best to seek expert help if your symptoms persist or worsen.

ADDITIONAL RESOURCES
Books and Publications:

1.**"The China Study"** by T. Colin Campbell and Thomas M. Campbell: Explores the relationship between the consumption of animal products and chronic illnesses.

2.**"Eat to Live"** by Joel Fuhrman, M.D.: Focuses on nutrient-dense, plant-rich eating for health and weight loss.

3.**"The Blue Zones"** by Dan Buettner: Investigates communities worldwide where people live longer and healthier lives.

4.**"Self Heal by Design"** by Barbara O'Neill: It embraces natural health principles and holistic practices for self-healing and wellness.

Printed in Great Britain
by Amazon

38280011R00056